Walking with the Genie

The Modern Woman's Menstrual Health Kit

BY ALEXANDRA POPE

First published in 2001 by
Alexandra Pope
PO Box 1018
Bondi Junction
NSW 1355
Australia

National Library of Australia Cataloguing-in-Publication entry:
Pope, A
Walking with the Genie: The modern woman's menstrual health kit

ISBN 0-9579614-0-5

Contents

1 Discovering the Power of Self Care

You too can reach menstrual wellbeing

Through the natural power of the menstrual cycle and by taking care of your overall health, you can reduce, or even eliminate, menstrual problems. Self care is the foundation for wellbeing – **you** taking responsibility for **your** health. Self care is your capacity to listen to, believe in and support yourself.

In this booklet I offer all women in their menstruating years a different way of thinking about menstruation. Reading this booklet will expand your understanding and help you maintain good health. I do not present you with a set of intractable rules. Rather, I encourage you to be open to the wisdom of your own being. Partners of women who suffer menstrual problems will also gain an insight into this wisdom.

Work with a natural health practitioner

If you suffer from menstrual problems, I suggest you also work with a natural health practitioner for guidance on what herbal and vitamin and mineral supplements to take. But always remember, this professional help is not a substitute for your ongoing self care.

Become curious

Pay attention to the subtleties of your experience – become like a detective hunting clues. Go to lots of different sources to gather information and ask lots of questions. It's particularly useful to talk to other women who suffer from similar problems – ask them about their experience of different therapeutic approaches.

Trust your own innate wisdom

Always remember that you're the one who has to live with your body – no one else! What might feel right for you may not look right to others. Consider carefully what others have to say, but always come back to what feels right for you, what **you** are ready for.

Listen to your symptoms

It's helpful to see symptoms as meaningful – otherwise you may end up feeling powerless and empty. Symptoms are a call to attend to your physical health. They are also a wise teacher helping you to become more thoughtful and sensitive towards yourself and the world. They could be a wake-up call encouraging you to express parts of yourself you normally don't. Like all disturbance they break the mould of your habitual way of operating and challenge you to do things differently. However, this doesn't mean that each symptom has a specific meaning that's true for all people. Each person's experience is unique.

Suffering makes us more vulnerable. Vulnerability is not a weakness, it's an opening. Initially it might feel overwhelming but if you're tender and kind with yourself you'll start to notice and feel different things about yourself and the world. It's important to pay attention to this – your capacity to allow yourself to be opened and changed is what makes symptoms meaningful. For example, instead of taking painkillers for your period pain, give in to it for a little while. Stop and rest. Just doing this will reveal feelings and ideas that seem to come out of nowhere.

Become difficult

It's the "difficult" person who heals. According to distinguished American surgeon Dr Bernie Siegel, the so-called "problem" patient is also the rapid healer, the one with the active immune system. "Difficult" people are only seen as difficult because they won't go along with the status quo – they aren't nice at the expense of themselves. They often speak difficult truths. If you're suffering from health problems you may already be perceived as "difficult". Worse still, changing your diet, taking a fiercer stand for your needs, not always being there for others in the way they're used to, may initially create discomfort for you and others. This doesn't mean that what you are doing is wrong – it's just different. So value difficultness – it's making you well!

Give yourself time

Some of the remedies I recommend are ones that quietly take effect over time. I encourage you to give yourself time to unfold your path of healing. Healing often involves a reorienting of your whole life and you may need to grow into things slowly – some things in life hate to be rushed. Nature, our bodies, our souls, intimacy and healing all have a pace vastly different from the fast paced existence that too many of us get caught up in today. You might be surprised at how the simple act of slowing down can produce remarkably quick results!

Invest wisely

Getting well can be an expensive business – the cost of regular visits to health practitioners and the various remedies such as herbs, homoeopathics, vitamins and minerals can become exorbitant over time. Eating well is also expensive. But to cut corners with your health while spending lavishly in other areas is a false economy. I encourage you to do the best you can according to your budget. Regard your health spending as an investment – with good health other things will flow, including your ability to increase your income. And remember, there are some practices such as rest, regular exercise and getting natural light which cost nothing!

2 Those Wayward Hormones

An early warning system

The menstrual cycle allows us to generate and regenerate. It gives women the possibility to create life. And all women, regardless of whether they suffer infertility, have the opportunity each month at menstruation to renew their own body and spirit.

The stress-sensitive system in women, the menstrual cycle is a self referencing and early warning system for your overall wellbeing. When problems arise within the cycle it's the body's way of encouraging you to pay attention to yourself. This is a gift. And as much as you might want to ignore your period pain by taking painkillers, or dismiss your premenstrual emotional upheavals as "just premenstrual", these and many other menstrual difficulties are giving you useful information about yourself: your overall health, the needs of your soul, the quality of your relationships and the environment in which you live. If you suffer from severe menstrual problems, it's likely your overall health is poor – the difficulties within the cycle alert you to this.

So it's important to listen to your body/self and to respect your experience even if you don't understand it. This takes courage, particularly in a culture that can still sometimes trivialise women's experience, especially around menstruation.

A woman who appreciates the nuances of her menstrual cycle can deepen knowledge of herself, build self esteem and develop a high sensitivity. She builds a unique form of strength and intelligence.

Understanding menstrual problems

Menstrual difficulties, like any other health problems, are linked to many factors including:

- poor diet
- stress
- poor digestion

- hypoglycaemia
- impaired immune system
- environmental pollution
- overweight or underweight
- hormonal imbalance
- congenital and hereditary weakness
- personal psychological trauma
- low self-esteem
- cultural devaluation of the feminine

They're all interconnected. For example, too much stress or a poor diet can weaken your immune system. Your hormones can be out of balance because of stress, a polluted environment and poor diet. You can feel bad about yourself because you're unwell or live or work in a discriminatory environment.

To heal and stay well you need to eat well, take regular exercise, minimize environmental pollution, nourish your soul, build self-esteem and have a sense of meaning in your life. These are all things you can do for yourself – they are practices for life.

You may also need to get support from a health practitioner. The following therapies could be beneficial for you:

- Acupuncture
- Homoeopathy
- Naturopathy
- Chiropractic
- Osteopathy
- Herbs: Chinese and Western
- Massage: remedial and shiastu
- Orthobionomy
- Reflexology
- Reiki
- Yoga
- Feldenkrais

- Tai Chi/Qi Gong
- Kinesiology
- Holographic Repatterning
- Counselling
- Psychodrama
- Art, music and dance therapy
- Spiritual healing
- Flower essences

Drugs and surgery

Regardless of whether you've already chosen the path of surgery and/or drugs, or are considering it, there are still a lot of other things you can do to improve your health and wellbeing. Drugs and surgery are an adjunct to self care - not a substitute.

If you haven't decided yet on drugs or surgery, you might want to try some of the practices in this booklet, and also explore alternative remedies, first. You'll need to allow yourself two to three months for the natural remedies to take effect. Make sure you tell your doctor what you're doing, particularly if you're taking vitamins or herbs and are considering surgery.

3 Some Great Natural Medicines

Become interested in the whole of your cycle

We are cyclical beings. Cycles are the basis of life – going against them is a recipe for disruption and possible sickness. We have different needs and tendencies at different phases of the cycle. This is normal and not a sign of weakness.

The more you start paying attention to your body, the more you will discover what needs healing and what is already improving. Attention itself is healing and being in touch with the rhythms of the body is empowering. You are cultivating the skill of self awareness.

Become aware of shifts in feeling and energy, the quality of your dreams and your needs throughout the cycle. Always have an idea of roughly when menstruation is due. For those of you with a regular cycle this is pretty easy.

You can chart your cycle in a more formal sense for contraception and conception purposes by recording cervical mucous, temperature and other body changes (for a detailed description of this, see *Natural Fertility* by Francesca Naish). For those of you with irregular cycles, still chart your cycle – you may even discover a pattern within the so-called irregularity!

- *Write in your diary the date when you're period is due.*
- *Make that a special time for you in some way, however small.*
- *Try doing nothing, or at least having some "nothing" time on that day.*

Support your tendencies

Much of our suffering comes from our inability to support our natural tendencies coming into, and during, menstruation. Learn to cooperate with yourself, rather than always imposing regimes and activities regardless of your changing needs and feelings. Cooperating as much as possible with your tendencies builds self esteem. It allows you to become responsive to the world, rather than reactive, thereby increasing your effectiveness.

Especially be aware of what you'd like to do around menstruation if you weren't worrying about the needs and expectations of others. What you come up with is the very thing you need to do! Even if you can only manage to do it briefly, it will make a difference to your sense of wellbeing. You might simply need more solitude, quiet time or to do less. If you feel the urge to retreat, retreat. If you become more vague, go more slowly, allow for some dreamy vague time, which has its own magic. At first it may feel strange to go against what you consider "normal" but, as you allow yourself to shift gear, other opportunities with open up to you.

- *Plan for what you would like at menstruation.*
- *Keep the diary empty of commitments around your period so there is space to follow your needs.*

Focus into yourself at menstruation

During the ovulatory phase of the cycle we are more outer focused – there for others, active and achieving "out there". As we move towards menstruation the spotlight moves off others and onto ourselves. This can be uncomfortable if we're not happy with our lives, if we are not used to focusing on ourselves, or our sense of purpose comes from "doing" for others.

The internal space of menstruation allows for self reflection and a greater capacity for feeling. All those reactive, vulnerable and complicated feelings associated with the premenstruum and menstruation are the clues to a deeper story in you wishing to be expressed. Don't ignore or trivialise these feelings! Women have a natural built-in reminder to attend to themselves. This is the regeneration process at work.

- *Ease back on being your usual generous self to the world and give some of that to yourself, especially if you're a mother.*
- *Say "no" more often.*
- *Practise tenderness with yourself, indulge, write in your journal, slob around.*
- *Don't go the extra mile for anyone, get them to do it for you.*
- *Practise being "gloriously selfish".*

Honour this time of high sensitivity

I bet some of you know feelings of high sensitivity all too well - all those messy, mushy, tender, reactive, angry, provocative feelings! At menstruation we move into a much more charged state emotionally. We literally become more open. To everything! What we might normally hold back on during the rest of the month may come bursting through at this time.

We're also more easily affected by what's around us. Unwittingly we may become the conduits for the unexpressed charge, or unacknowledged feelings, in people around us (particularly our partners, children and work colleagues). Yes, we can actually feel for the world as well.

While your feelings might feel horrible, embarrassing or something to be ashamed of, they are your life blood. They are what make you human – without them life would have no meaning. Unfortunately we can't take the nice bits and leave the nasty ones out. It's the whole package or nothing at all! Feelings are a way of "knowing" about the world. Without feelings it's impossible to make fully informed and wise decisions.

If you find the menstrual sensitivity just too overwhelming, and perhaps even faint, you may be a sensitive – a highly intuitive person who has an ability to "see into things", a psychic. To you, the world can feel invasive. If you ignore your talent for sensitivity it may turn up as distress and distressing symptoms. But as you accommodate it, the sensitivity will feel less like a liability and more like a wonderful heightened state of awareness allowing you access to a more expanded reality.

- *Begin to cultivate a curiosity for the different currents of feeling moving through you.*
- *Understand that all your feelings are meaningful and not always personal.*
- *If you have trouble trying to unfold that meaning or to stand up for what you feel, consider seeing a counsellor or psychotherapist to assist you.*
- *Learn to be more protective of yourself in the premenstruum if you do find yourself overwhelmed with strong emotion.*
- *If you are a sensitive, protect yourself – give space and time for your talent by stepping out of regular life for a little while.*
- *Take time alone, enjoying silence (no TV, no computers, no phones, no newspapers!), resting, drifting, dreaming, following whims, meditating.*

Nurture your relationships

Menstruation can be an amazing ally or a great disturber in relationships – often a bit of both! This disturbance can potentially strengthen the relationship and the vulnerability at menstruation can be an opening to deeper intimacy. The key is to be aware of your tendencies and needs. And to feel comfortable asserting those needs. It also depends on how comfortable your partner is with him or herself and their willingness to be open to change. All these can grow with time and care – menstruation is your training ground for deepening the relationship.

Let your partner know what you prefer to do at, or leading into, menstruation. He or she is not a mind reader! Enlist their support, knowing that what you ask for you are quite happy to offer to your partner in return at another time of the month.

If you find yourself becoming very picky, reactive or highly critical of your partner in the premenstruum, pay attention to these grievances. The premenstruum is categorically **not** a time to abuse anyone, yourself included. But it can be a time for some straight talking. Ideally, I would encourage you to deal with these issues during the rest of the month rather than waiting for menstruation. If you're not skilled at using the charge of this time you might be slightly less than diplomatic!!

Sometimes the premenstrual reactivity is simply an unrecognised need for time out from having to attend to or be mindful of others. The menstruating woman may also unwittingly become the channel of expression for what her partner is failing to express – don't assume that the reactivity is all "her stuff". It's equally important that husbands/lovers don't dismiss their menstruating partner's moods as "just premenstrual" – this trivialises a very real experience and exacerbates the distress. The feelings are meaningful, it just takes time sometimes to work out what's going on.

- *Communicate!*
- *Take tender "down time" together at menstruation.*
- *Encourage your partner to join you in some of your health practices – they are just good healthy practices for anyone.*
- *Encourage your partner to familiarise him or herself with the information in this booklet.*
- *Use menstruation as a time for quietness together, an opportunity to deepen intimacy.*

Get in touch with the power of menstruation

Menstruation is a highly charged state, a natural high where intuition, psychic skills and dreaming are more developed. It's a window of opportunity, a time for visioning, creativity, wisdom, insight, prayer, ritual and magic. It's a place to garner soul food and guidance for your life. What a pity to waste these amazing strengths by continuing on the same as before!

Think of your premenstrual unsettledness as a wise voice reminding you it's time to tune into those strengths. In some indigenous cultures the menstruating woman was seen as the truth speaker for her community. Your premenstrual "aggressive" outbursts could be an honest punchy declaration that needs to be heard.

The first day or two of the period is a great letting go and clearing out time, followed by a space of extraordinary clarity, a clarity which may elude you if you don't let yourself have some time for really letting go.

- *Give yourself a completely empty space to do nothing and notice what arises in you!*
- *Meditate and create ritual.*
- *Use menstruation as a moment for visioning for future projects or even the coming month.*
- *Speak challenging truths.*
- *When you have a major life decision to make, instead of "sleeping" on it, allow yourself to "bleed" on the problem. If you have the time, give yourself one cycle to feel and think into the issue, and as you bleed watch what arises from within.*

Slow down

By now you should be getting the message that slowing down is a good thing at menstruation. Resting may be all the remedy that most of us need! Time to do nothing.

This may feel like the end of the world to the active busy part of yourself. Doing nothing is often seen as a waste of time. Wanting to be alone can be seen as antisocial and therefore a sign that something is "wrong" with you. Throw all that thinking out! Rest and alone time are essential for the body and soul. If you feel the need for it that's a good enough reason. Whether we are highly sensitive or not, we all have an ability to enter an expanded reality, another world of experience, at menstruation. Being still allows this to happen.

If you suffer from period pain, try rest instead of painkillers. Resting alone can ease pain, and over time primary dysmenorrhoea (painful periods) may ease altogether. Many premenstrual symptoms also improve with plenty of rest, sleep and extra dreaming time.

Exercise regularly

Many of the classic menstrual symptoms are about stuck energy, including bloating, constipation, depression, irritability and cramping. Exercise will literally help to "move things". Choose exercise that you feel drawn to and avoid "punishing" your body. This work is all about being in tune with your body, not giving it a hard time! Try yoga, walking, swimming (avoid chlorinated pools), tai chi/qi gong, Feldenkrais, rebounding, dancing (especially belly dancing), working out at a gym, or any sport that gives you pleasure.

Poor body structure can contribute to period pain. Practices such as yoga and tai chi are particularly useful for improving body structure, as well as strengthening and energising the body. You may also benefit from receiving some body work such as shiatsu, remedial massage, osteopathy and chiropractic.

Reduce stress

Too much stress is bad news for your health. Remember, the menstrual cycle is your stress-sensitive system. That means it's like a barometer for how you're handling things generally. It's critical to find ways of reducing the stress in your life.

Sometimes when we're highly stressed we may not have been standing up for ourselves enough. In these economically rationalised times, some work environments have also become very stressful from too much work and less job security. While stress management and relaxation techniques are useful, you may also need to change the situations that are causing you stress, rather than trying to make yourself fit into the stressful situation.

It may help to seek support from a counsellor to build your self esteem. Sometimes the solutions needed are political. For example, it may be important to join a union to fight for fairer wages and conditions.

Stop smoking and avoid passive smoking

This is essential. If you're a smoker, and this includes marijuana, I recommend you make quitting a priority. Try your local community health centre or health fund for a "Stop Smoking" programme. Also consider acupuncture, hypnotherapy, 12 step groups and counselling.

Read inspiring books on menstruation

The history of menstruation is rich and complex, and snakes back to the very origins of culture. The loss of this history sustains a climate of secrecy and shame in our natural body processes. For those of you who suffer at menstruation it can be doubly humiliating. Recover some of this knowledge and re-empower yourself.

4 Healthy Spaces

The impact of environmental pollution on our health is enormous. Your endometriosis, fibroid, excessive blood, pain, premenstrual anguish and polycystic ovaries are all directly linked to increasing environmental pollution. Through everyday exposure to toxic chemicals and electromagnetic radiation, our body's ability to repair itself is being seriously zapped.

There are toxic chemicals in the water we drink and the food we buy. There are chemicals in household cleaners, pest sprays, clothes, furnishings, paints, plastics, skin and hair products, makeup, perfumes, books, newspapers and magazines. Outside the home we have pollution from cars and trucks, aeroplanes, polluting industries and chemicalised agribusiness.

We are exposing ourselves to radiation pollution in the everyday technology we use, such as microwave ovens, televisions, computers and mobile phones and other electrical devices – even seemingly harmless appliances like hairdryers and electric clocks. Radiation also comes from x-rays, high voltage power lines and flying in aeroplanes.

In some workplaces there's a high use of chemicals – if you're a hairdresser, photographer, beautician, agricultural worker, chemical worker, textile and leather worker or if you work in the car manufacturing and repair industry you will be exposed to toxic chemicals. Those working with electronics and semiconductors, food workers, workers in manufacturing and printing, glass and pottery, and hospital and health care staff are also all at risk.

Skin and hair products are a minefield of synthetic chemicals. Most of the chemicals that go into our toiletries are also the harsh toxic chemicals used in industry. For example, propylene glycol, found in makeup, hair care products, deodorants and aftershave, is also the main ingredient in antifreeze and brake fluid. Polyethylene glycol, found in most skin cleansers, is a caustic used to dissolve grease (Thomas, 1999).

The accumulative effect of all these environmental stressors plays havoc with human physiology, including your immune system and therefore your overall health. Other effects include cancer, infertility, birth defects and stillbirths (Naish and Roberts, 1996).

To heal and maintain wellbeing it's essential to minimise pollutants in our personal life and attend to the environment as a whole. You'll be doing yourself an enormous favour and you'll also end up helping family, friends and co-workers.

You might also feel inspired to take bigger steps that involve support for environmental organisations, social action or a reorganisation of your whole life based on more sustainable practices. Regardless of whether you suffer health problems or not, the following points are a starting place to make changes in your personal environment.

Food

- Avoid canned food and plastic packaging. At the very least remove food from the packaging as soon as possible.
- Store food in glass containers.
- Use cloth and paper bags for storing vegetables.
- Try cellophane bags for storing or short term freezing only.
- Avoid aluminium and copper cookware, and avoid cooking or storing food in aluminium foil.
- Ideally use glass cookware.
- Avoid tetra packs which are lined with aluminium.
- Don't microwave your food. It's especially critical that you don't microwave children's food. Food that has been cooked or defrosted in a microwave can cause changes in the blood. This process is indicative of similar processes found in cancer (Best, 2000).
- Only drink or cook with filtered water, ideally filtered using the reverse osmosis system.
- Never eat processed breakfast cereals (they contain solvent remnants) and avoid processed foods wherever possible.
- Eat organic and biodynamic foods, and avoid genetically modified and irradiated food.

Your body

- Stop and think before you pile on skin care products – the skin absorbs everything so it's as good as eating it. And of course in the case or lipstick you literally are!
- Use plant-based beauty products, including perfumes, rather than petrochemically based ones. Listing some natural ingredients doesn't mean the product is all natural – so beware.
- Read labels carefully. Avoid ingredients such as sodium lauryl/laureth sulfate, talc, mineral oil, aluminium, glycol, and ones containing the letters "prop" e.g. propyl, propamine, isopropyl, propanol and propylene.
- Telephone the manufacturer and ask them to explain the ingredients and where they come from.
- Avoid using foundation as it prevents your skin breathing.
- Use toothpaste that is free of fluoride, sugar and sodium lauryl sulphate.
- Avoid hair dyes, especially dark colours.
- Use only biodegradable low allergenic formula washing powders and washing-up liquids free of unnecessary colourings and fragrances.
- Avoid having your clothes dry cleaned. If you must have this done, air the item of clothing outside for three days afterwards before wearing it.
- Avoid antiperspirants and deodorants, especially those containing aluminium. If you wear natural fibres you'll sweat less. Body odour will also decrease as you clean up your diet and lifestyle. The best underarm deodoriser is a dusting of plain old bicarbonate of soda. If the powder stings or burns, it means it has been contaminated during manufacture and should be thrown out and replaced with a different brand.
- Avoid mercury fillings. You could consider having existing mercury fillings removed – make sure this is done by a dentist fully versed in the protocol and who has a completely mercury-free practice. Having your amalgam fillings removed is not a procedure to enter into lightly although it may be necessary if your health is very poor. Read widely and ask questions before you make a decision.
- Avoid x-rays.
- Avoid oral contraceptives and wearing IUDs.
- Minimise or avoid using tampons especially if you suffer period pain.

Your home

- Use only "green" cleaning products. Check logos to ensure they have been tested and validated by the appropriate government agency.
- For all general cleaning and laundry, try old fashioned products such as bicarbonate of soda for sinks, refrigerators, baths and toilets. White vinegar can be used as a disinfectant.
- Avoid all pesticides but if you do need a thorough pest proofing of your home, use only pyrethrum-type compounds.
- Practice co-existence with insect life where possible. Put all food away and keep surfaces clean. To get rid of cockroaches try leaving out a bowl of beer - they'll at least die happy!
- You can buy non-toxic pest control products, including treatment for animal fleas. If you have a flea infestation, vacuum thoroughly for ten consecutive days, replace the vacuum bag each time, throwing out the used one right away.
- If you need a pest exterminator, contract an ecologically sound one. They will often be able to give you advice about safely minimising pests in your home.
- Keep soft plastic out of your life as much as possible, e.g. plastic bags of any kind, cling film, bubble wrap. Check every cupboard, it's surprising how much can be lurking. Also check the boot and inside of your car.
- Avoid aerosols and propellent sprays of any kind.
- Avoid cooking on gas, or using gas heaters, and consider changing to electric.
- Keep your home well aired at all times, especially the bathroom, to prevent build up of mould.
- Have live plants throughout the house to absorb pollution.
- Use a chlorine filter on the bath and shower heads, particularly the latter. You can absorb much more chlorine through breathing in the steam than through drinking.
- Use ionisers, especially at night when sleeping. Place the ioniser close to an open window to blow the negative ions through the room. Or buy two and place on either side of the bed. For maximum effect have several ionisers in the one room.
- When doing any renovations only use ecologically sound products (paint, stripper, varnishes) and beware of breathing in dust from the renovations.

- If you have a choice avoid carpets, enjoy (naturally!) polished wooden floors with rugs made from natural fibres.
- Avoid burning candles or incense.
- If you're a keen gardener, learn about organic and permaculture techniques to avoid use of pesticides, herbicides. Your garden will be healthier and happier as well!

Your workplace

- Learn basic information about workplace chemicals and their toxic effects.
- Meticulously follow all safety precautions.
- Keep workspaces as well ventilated as possible.
- Consider changing your job if the workplace is unhealthy.
- Use ionisers and live plants - the peace lily and spider plant absorb air pollution well, particularly around computers.
- Don't stand over photocopiers when they're in use.

City living

- If you own a car, use it less often to minimise your contribution to air pollution.
- If you drive, avoid heavy traffic, tunnels and using underground or enclosed parking.
- Keep windows closed in heavy traffic and enclosed areas.
- Consider using an ioniser in the car.
- Minimise how frequently you fill your car with petrol and try to avoid breathing in the fumes as much as possible.
- Avoid exercising in heavy traffic areas.
- Avoid other people's cigarette smoke and perfumes.

Electro magnetic radiation (EMR)

- Don't keep an electric clock by your bed as the EMR is very strong.
- Avoid electric blankets, or if you must have one, switch it off before going to sleep.
- Avoid hair dryers.
- Unplug all appliances that are not in use.

- Avoid locating beds and chairs close to domestic sources of EMR such as electricity meters and televisions.
- Use an ioniser especially when working at a computer. Either place the ioniser at eye level on top of the computer or buy two and put them on either side of you for a stereophonic effect. Never use just one ioniser on one side of you, as it will unbalance the body.
- Place plants around your computer, especially the spider plant and peace lily.
- Have regular epsom salt baths to help "cleanse" yourself of the effects of EMRs. Have plenty of contact with nature and the earth, even touching the plants in your office.
- Move away from your computer screen when involved in other activities.
- Turn off your computer when not in use.
- Try sipping water throughout the day, especially if you work at a computer or other electronic equipment.

5 The Joy of Good Food

A good diet is vital for wellbeing – no medication can overcome the effects of a poor diet. So regard healthy eating as an essential medicine for healing all menstrual problems. Food also gives us enormous pleasure and pleasure is essential to good health. Changing your diet doesn't mean you have to give up pleasure, it's just that the pleasures may change. With your new diet, you may find yourself enjoying the sensational taste of real food. You might actually like the sense of wellbeing you experience. You'll probably be delirious at being free from period pain! Rather than focusing on what you're giving up, think about what you're moving into to heal your body – the reward is a more vibrant and healthy lifestyle.

Although each person's needs are unique, and no one diet fits everyone, I will give you some useful guidelines. As food is a highly emotive issue for many people, particularly those of you who have battled with diets over the years, it's important to tread carefully and lightly with yourself in exploring the following health instructions.

If you're a woman who has had a history of anorexia, bulimia or binge eating, or if you're currently experiencing any of these, I suggest that diet is not the starting place for your menstrual healing work. If you're not already working with a psychotherapist, or belong to a support group, I recommend you start now. Making peace with yourself and your body will do wonders for your menstrual problems without even getting into managing food – an area for you that might be fraught with difficulty.

Many women ask me how long they have to be on the diet. A difficult question to answer because I would never recommend going back to a poor diet! However, as your health improves, you may enjoy foods on the "to avoid" list now and then. How you feel in your body will always be your guide – if your overall health is poor you may have to be much stricter with yourself.

As a general rule you need to give yourself at least three months on your new diet to allow for any health changes. Give yourself longer, say five or six months, if you're a bit on again/off again with the diet. No matter how small the changes you've made to your diet, you may have days when you can't do it. This is perfectly normal, so don't beat yourself up for eating inappropriate foods – enjoy eating them and then continue again the next day with the healthier plan. Do it consciously, rather than as a furtive reaction to that "damn diet". My only word of caution – try not to break the health rules in the few days before and during your period.

It's OK to grow into the changes slowly. Start with those parts of the diet you feel you can handle. Success will breed success. It's also fine if you're someone who likes to leap into the deep end, doing everything at once. You need to be aware, however, that when beginning a healing diet you may have what's known as a "healing crisis". This means you can feel worse before you feel better. You may get headaches, feelings of nausea or fatigue. Slowly introducing the health changes is a way to minimise this discomfort. If it does occur drink plenty of water, try gentle exercise or yoga, and get plenty of rest. It will pass and then you'll start to feel so much better.

Changing your diet can be disruptive to personal, work and family life. Because of this some women find the changes a little overwhelming, particularly if family and friends don't take your condition seriously. Move with caution but never give up on your quest for wellbeing. Asking those close to you to read this booklet may also help. It's important to note the health changes I recommend are generally beneficial for everyone. Your loved ones might be happy to join you in some of them!

A healthy digestive system

You need wonderful digestion for wonderful health. A healthy digestive system is as critical for wellbeing as good food. If your digestion is poor you won't be able to absorb all the nutrients – even if you eat the best food in the world! Chances are you'll also not be eliminating wastes from the body very well either. This means a build up of toxins further hindering wellbeing.

Women with menstrual problems usually have some digestive disturbance. If you have any kind of chronic digestive disturbance such as wind, bloating, pain, chronic constipation, diarrhoea, or irregular bowel movements, you may need to seek professional help along with making healthy changes in your diet. If you don't attend to these problems you'll see little improvement – I can't emphasis this enough.

Constipation and other digestive difficulties can worsen period pain. If you have a tendency to constipation, eat plenty of vegies, fruit, including apricots and prunes, ground linseed and calcium rich foods (calcium aids peristalsis). Drink plenty of water and avoid junk and processed foods. Take regular exercise, especially before breakfast, as well as getting plenty of natural light (see page 38). Castor oil and linseed packs may also help. If none of these bring you joy, do seek professional support from a practitioner well versed in natural health.

If you're on the Pill, take painkillers each month to manage your menstrual pain, or other drugs to manage endometriosis, be aware that you can adversely affect your digestive system, and therefore in the long term undermine your efforts for menstrual wellbeing.

Allergies are a sign that your immune system is not functioning well. Allergies have a talent for masking themselves as other illnesses. For example, your period pain could be connected to a particular food substance. The most common ones are pasteurised/homogenised, inorganic cow's milk, wheat, eggs, yeast and dust mites. Alternative therapies such as naturopathy, homoeopathy, chiropractic, acupuncture and Chinese herbs can help enormously.

Foods that promote health

An important aspect of overcoming menstrual health problems is to become an aware consumer. Read labels carefully and avoid all foods with additives, colourings or genetically engineered ingredients. The best way to ensure you're getting healthy food is to buy organic, biodynamic or grow your own.

The following are some foods that will help you enormously in your quest for menstrual health and general wellbeing.

Whole foods and minimally processed foods. Examples of whole foods are brown rice rather than white rice, brown flour rather than white flour. Minimally processed foods include tofu and fermented foods such as miso and yoghurt.

Fresh food. I have a contract with myself not to eat food that's more than a day old. For example, I might make enough dinner so there's some left over for a lunch box the next day, but if I haven't eaten it by then I throw it away. It's important to avoid food that has gone mouldy, particularly if you have allergies. Remember to enjoy foods in season.

Organically and biodynamically produced food. Organically and biodynamically produced food is much tastier and contains more vitamins and minerals than conventionally produced food. Most importantly, it doesn't contain the pesticides, chemical fertilisers, growth hormones, antibiotics and vaccines that regular fruit, vegetables, meat, eggs and dairy products contain. Avoid genetically engineered food at all times. Buying certified organic food is one way to ensure you're not eating genetically engineered food.

The greatest possible variety. You're more likely to get the range of nutrients your body needs if you have a varied diet. You're also less likely to develop an allergy which can occur if you repeatedly eat the same foods.

Vegetables. Most vegies are rich in vitamins and minerals. Particularly good ones for women with menstrual problems are root vegies and the green leafy varieties. Make fresh vegetables the mainstay of your diet.

Whole grains and whole grain cereal. These include brown rice, corn, oats, rye, millet, buckwheat, quinoa, amaranth and wheat. Wheat can worsen bloating and gas, a sign that you could be allergic to it. In your quest for menstrual health, I would even go so far as to say that wheat may be one of the foods you consider giving up first.

Legumes. These include lentils, kidney beans, azuki beans, chick peas, haricot beans, lima beans, black-eyed beans, black beans, split peas.

Seeds and nuts. Avoid peanuts and peanut butter, as well as pistachios, as they usually contain mould. Unlike meat and fish, beans, nuts and seeds are not complete proteins. However, by coupling them with a grain, you have a complete protein. You don't need to eat them in the same meal to get the benefit of the protein. It's important to store nuts, seeds, and their spreads, in the refrigerator to prevent them from becoming rancid. Eat nuts and seeds within a few weeks of purchase and only buy from shops where there's a high turnover of stock. Avoid stale nuts and seeds at all costs.

Fruits. Enjoy fruits that are seasonal. Fresh fruit is a good source of vitamins and fibre.

Oils. Use only cold-pressed, unrefined oils. Olive (virgin only) and sesame are the best for everyday use. Avoid canola oil. Ideally buy oils in brown bottles, to minimise the deteriorating effects of light, and keep them in the refrigerator. Don't even think about buying the de-odourised, sanitised (hydrogenated) versions you find in supermarkets. Hydrogenation creates an immune damaging fat so these oils have no goodness left in them and may even be bad for you.

Essential fatty acids (EFAs). Essential for good health, EFAs are particularly important for women with menstrual problems. We need them for the formation of the "friendly" prostaglandins that help to ease cramping.

Particularly rich sources of EFAs are flaxseed (linseed), evening primrose oil, walnuts, raw goat's milk and the oil in fatty fish. Enjoy freshly ground linseed sprinkled on your food as an economical and easy way to get these nutrients.

Tofu. Made from soy beans, tofu is a good protein source. Soy beans are a source of plant oestrogens which may help relieve PMS symptoms by competing with your own level of oestrogen when it's too high. Tofu is not fermented, so if you have severe health problems or very poor digestion, avoid eating it.

Shoyu or tamari. These are fermented soy products made from water, salt and soya beans. Use as a salt substitute as they contain much less sodium.

Miso. A fermented soya bean paste, miso contains protein and helps fight fatigue. It's a great aid to digestion – as long as you don't boil the paste – and a good salt substitute.

Tempeh. An Indonesian food, tempeh is fermented soy beans (again!). It's very nutritious and an excellent protein product. Although an acquired taste for some people, it's worthwhile learning some tasty recipes.

Seaweeds. A powerhouse of minerals, vitamins and amino acids, seaweeds are an excellent source of iodine, calcium and iron in an easily assimilated form. Never mind diamonds being a girl's best friend, minerals are – seaweeds are a great way to ensure you get plenty of them! Seaweeds will help prevent damage to tissues from chemicals, heavy metals, and certain types of radioactivity; offset stress, boost stamina, and restore sexual interest (Weed, 1989). Types of seaweed include nori, arame, kombu, wakame and Tasmanian float leaf. You can also buy kelp seaweed in tablet and powdered form, using the latter as a salt substitute if you wish.

Water. Essential for all chemical processes in your body, water also helps memory and flushes toxins from the body. I suspect that premenstrual headaches have a lot to do with dehydration. Start drinking more water from today, particularly in hot weather or if you exercise heavily. Because of the many chemicals used in our water supply, a water filter is essential. A reverse osmosis filter system is the best, but initially buy whatever you can afford. Or buy bottled water in clear plastic or glass bottles only.

The great soy debate

Although soy products, such as tofu and soy milk, are frequently touted as a great source of protein, and a panacea for the woes of menopause, some health practitioners believe soy products are too difficult to digest and should be avoided. Another complication is that soy beans were one of the first foods to be genetically engineered and for this reason alone I would encourage you to eat only organic or bio-dynamic soy.

The specific soy products I recommend are prepared using traditional methods such as soaking, long slow cooking and natural fermentation and are therefore OK. Other modern soy food, such as milk, cheese, and soy protein isolates used in some soy milks, protein supplements, baby formulas and many "instant" packaged foods, are prepared in high tech, high speed ways that denature the food. Research has found that these products are difficult to digest and can lead to deficiencies of zinc, calcium, B12, and vitamins A and D.

It's not necessary to eat soy products to have a healthy diet. If you don't like them don't force yourself. Listen to your body on this one!

The following table will help you work out specific ways to improve your diet. The foods listed in the "avoid or reduce" column are those foods that worsen menstrual health. Following the recommendations is particularly important if you experience menstrual symptoms; however, they are also useful for those women wishing to maintain wellbeing.

Avoid or reduce	Alternative
Dairy products: cow's milk and cheese, butter and butter spreads, yoghurt. (Note: women not experiencing menstrual difficulties can enjoy organic dairy products). **Problem:** • Dairy products create a watery, bloated feeling or edema. This can worsen candida, and is implicated in a prolapsed uterus. • Dairy products interfere with the absorption of magnesium, a mineral which is helpful for easing menstrual cramps, stabilising blood sugar levels and mood swings. • They contribute to the production of series 2 prostaglandins (hormone like substances in the body) the "baddies" implicated in menstrual cramping. The "good" prostaglandins, series 1 and 3, which ease pain, are created by eating the healthy diet described here.	• *Enjoy fermented organic and biodynamic products, such as yoghurt and cheese, that use unhomogenised milk.* • *Eat small amounts of goat's and sheep's milk products which are easier to digest than cow's. Unpasteurised goat's milk is also full of live enzymes, a nourishing food that's more easily tolerated than other dairy products.* • *Rice, almond or oat milk are good substitutes for cow's milk.* • *Consider coming off dairy products altogether for at least three months, particularly if you have endometriosis. Later you may be able to enjoy them.* • *Use seed and nut butter (e.g. tahini), and virgin olive oil instead of butter.* ***Don't*** *even consider margarine – throw out any tubs you have lurking in the fridge now.*

<table>
<tr><th>Avoid or reduce</th><th>Alternative</th></tr>
<tr><td>
Yeasted breads and bakery products: commercial cakes, biscuits and pastries.
Problem:
<ul>
<li>Yeast contributes to candida</li>
<li>White flour acidifies the body and in turn leaches it of minerals</li>
<li>Often made using hydrogenated oils.</li>
</ul>
</td><td>
<ul>
<li>Eat organic sourdough wholewheat bread. Some sourdoughs may contain a little yeast, so read the label carefully.</li>
<li>Even better, try a wheat-free sourdough bread or rice cakes.</li>
<li>Minimise your consumption of breads, pasta and cakes altogether, and replace with small amounts of whole grains such as rice or millet.</li>
<li>If life without cakes and cookies feels too miserable, try your health food store for the occasional sweet treat – naturally sweetened, and using cold pressed oils or butter. Although butter is on the "to avoid" list because it's too rich for your liver, it's much safer than the trans-fat/ hydrogenated oils and is therefore preferable. Consider making your own sweet treats from one of the many excellent wholefood cookery books on the market.</li>
</ul>
</td></tr>
</table>

Avoid or reduce	Alternative
Meat: beef, organ meats such as liver and kidneys, pork, lamb, chicken and meat products such as sausages or hot dogs, and all deli meats which may contain nitrate preservatives. **Problem:** • Opinions vary on meat. Some health experts say all meat is bad, while others say we do need a little. • Meat is difficult to digest and may lead to worsened pain and PMS. • Non-organically produced meat is full of toxins from antibiotics, vaccines, hormones and pesticides. The chemicals in our environment get transported in the food chain through animal fats. • Too much meat increases the body's demand for minerals.	• *I suggest eating meat no more than three times a week. Giving it up altogether even for a short time may be necessary for some of you, particularly if you have endometriosis and general cramping.* • *Always eat lots of vegetables and fruit if you eat meat.* • *At the very least don't eat animal fat.* • *If you do eat meat, only eat organically produced meat.* • *Eat instead deep ocean fish and occasional organic free-range chicken. Don't even look at battery chicken except to take a stance for stopping the inhumane treatment of these birds.* • *It's essential to only eat organ meats that are organically produced.* • *Only ever eat organic free-range eggs.* • *Chicken soup made from the bones is also very nourishing.* • *Don't forget the great vegetable sources of protein mentioned.*

Avoid or reduce	Alternative
Caffeinated drinks (coffee, tea and cola drinks), decaffeinated coffee **Problem:** • Caffeine depletes the body of B vitamins. • It contributes to anxiety and irritability and worsens mood swings. • Decaffeinated coffee contains solvents and even if it's water processed there are other inflammatory alkaloids. • Caffeine may have an adverse effect on your fertility.	• *Unroasted or roasted dandelion root coffee is good for the liver and digestion.* • *Grain-based beverages, such as Caro or Ecco are safe substitutes for coffee.* • *Ginger tea is excellent for fatigue. Bancha tea with a drop of shoyu and some grated ginger is also a great pick-me-up.* • *Try also the wide variety of herbal teas. The mineral-rich nettle tea is good for the kidneys and adrenals (the glands that sit on top of your kidneys and form part of your endocrine system) – a true friend to women!*

Avoid or reduce	Alternative
Alcohol **Problem:** • Alcohol depletes the body of minerals and B vitamins. • It's toxic to the liver. • It makes candida worse.	• *Drink no more than two glasses of wine, diluted with mineral water, a week.* • *Fresh vegetable or fruit juice. Go very easy on fruit juice as it has a high sugar content – dilute it with purified water or mineral water.* • *Consider giving up alcohol altogether and develop the water drinking habit.*

Avoid or reduce	Alternative
Refined sugar (sucrose), cane sugar, molasses, artificial sweeteners, soft drinks **Problem:** • Sucrose and artificial sweeteners, such as aspartamine, nutrasweet and saccharin, are "empty" foods – they have no nutrient value and are potentially bad for you. Sugar enters the blood stream too quickly, upsetting your blood sugar levels, stressing your adrenals. In the long run refined sugar makes you more fatigued and depletes you of minerals and B complex vitamins. It also contributes to premenstrual crankiness and fatigue. As your overall diet improves you may find your sugar cravings decrease. • Soft drinks are full of either refined sugar or artificial sweeteners and are to be avoided all costs. Far from quenching your thirst they will dehydrate your body. • The more sugar you eat, the more you will crave it.	• *Use rice or barley malt and sugar-free jams.* • *Use stevia, a very sweet herb, in place of sugar.* • *Pear or apple juice concentrate, and dried fruits such as dates, are good baking sweeteners as the natural sugar enters the blood stream more slowly and therefore is much gentler on the body.* • *Complex carbohydrates such as brown rice, wholemeal bread and oats can reduce your sugar craving. Try also baked pumpkin and sweet potato.* • *Honey and maple syrup as a very occasional treat are OK if you're desperate!*

Avoid or reduce	Alternative
Chocolate **Problem:** • Chocolate contains refined sugar, which contributes to mood swings and breast tenderness. It also contains caffeine. • Because it contains magnesium (good for cramping and mood swings) and the mood enhancer amino acid phenylalanine, you can understand why you might have such an intense craving just before bleeding. Alas, the other ingredients preclude it as a helpful food source!	• *Unsweetened carob is a member of the legume family and high in calcium. You can buy carob in chunk form as a substitute for a chocolate bar or as a powder to use in baking and drinks. Beware - some brands of carob "chocolate" contain sugar. Avoid these! Read the labels carefully – there are some tasty brands that don't contain sugar.* • *Although organic choc is still chocolate, it has a lot more going for it than the regular stuff. And it's expensive which may act as tiny brake on overindulgence! The* ***odd*** *mouthful in those chocolate crises may do a lot for your psyche without too much upset to your body.*

Avoid or reduce	Alternative
Free-flowing salt and high sodium foods (bouillon, commercial salad dressings and tomato sauces, salty snack foods) **Problem:** • These foods worsen bloating and fluid retention. • Regular free flowing salt bought in supermarkets contains additives – so avoid it! • The added sugar, hydrogenated oils, preservatives and food colouring in commercial sauces, dressings and snack foods are just further flak for your body to deal with.	• *You may need a little salt – I recommend mineral rich coarse sea salt from your health food shop. It looks grey and lumpy, and will definitely not flow through your salt shaker!* • *Try seasoning your foods with herbs, a little shoyu or miso.* • *You can buy good quality tomato sauce, mayonnaise and dressings, without additives, at health food shops – always check labels carefully.*

Making life easier

- Think about adding new foods to your diet before removing the less supportive ones.
- If you eat a lot of the foods on the "avoid" list, **don't** come off them suddenly.
- Change one thing at a time. Start with what's easiest for you, e.g. drinking more water.
- Relax and enjoy what you eat while being honest with yourself and tuning into your body's specific needs. If you run on a diet of coffee and sugar, both addictive substances, it will take you a little time to identify your body's genuine needs from an addictive craving.
- Be especially careful about sticking to the healthy diet in the second half of your menstrual cycle, particularly the week before you bleed and during bleeding.
- Make sure you have plenty of nutritious but tasty snacks available at all times to stop the "munchies" from forcing you down to the corner shop.
- Don't shop when you're hungry.
- Get a good wholefood, sugar-free recipe book and/or go to some health oriented cookery lessons. Any new diet can be time consuming, and some of the ingredients of the ones I have recommended take time to prepare – beans and grains will not be hurried!
- Chew your food really well. The first stage of digestion, in particular with carbohydrates, begins in the mouth. The action of chewing also helps to stimulate hydrochloric acid in the stomach which is essential for protein digestion.
- Eat when you're feeling calm. If you're upset, wait until your feelings have settled.
- Although some oil in the diet is necessary, avoid fried and oily foods, particularly around menstruation.
- Avoid extremely hot or extremely cold food as it may cause indigestion.
- At menstruation, eat lightly and prepare easily digestable foods such as soups, especially if you suffer period pain. For example, one pot "soupy" dishes with some grain, vegies and some beans or a little fish simmered together for a while with the addition of some herbs or a little fresh ginger is perfect.

- Eat defrosted food that you've prepared yourself, rather than packaged pre-prepared food. This is infinitely preferable to finding yourself starving and rushing out for pizza because there's nothing easy on hand to prepare.
- Avoid aluminium and copper cookware – use only glass or stainless steel.
- Minimise use of canned food.
- Always read labels assiduously – you need to become your own watch-dog. Avoid all foods containing synthetic colouring and additives.

To eat raw food or not?

Traditional Chinese Medicine does not recommend eating raw food the week before and during menstruation. It takes more energy to digest and is cooling on the body. Of course, eating foods that cool the body is, for instance, important during the hot days of summer. However, generally when we menstruate, and particularly if we have problems, eating more "warming", easily digestible foods is, overall, very nourishing and supportive for the body.

In the Western naturopathic traditions, raw food is seen as A Good Thing. I have come from a macrobiotic (Asian) approach to food, where everything is cooked. Today I'm drawn to the Western naturopathic model – I eat at least 75 per cent of my diet as raw food and feel fantastic. Cooking destroys enzymes which are essential for health. Listen to your own instincts on what feels right to you. Lightly cooking the food does not destroy all its nutrients.

6 More Ways to Pamper Yourself

Use cloth pads, sea sponges and organic tampons

If you're a die-hard tampon user, only use organic cotton tampons. Ideally minimise use of tampons. Avoid tampons altogether if you suffer period pain, heavy bleeding, fibroids or pelvic inflammatory disease (PID).

If your flow is not too heavy, try a sea sponge. Before you use the sponge, soak it in purified water. After use wash the sponge thoroughly and rinse in a vinegar/purified water solution. Dry in the sun.

Reusable cloth pads are much kinder to the body and the environment than tampons and disposable pads. They're easy to care for (instructions come with the pads) and you'll never run out – saving money in the long run! Quite a few women have observed they also bleed less with cloth pads. I cannot explain this phenomenon; however, if you do bleed excessively do give them a try.

If you're a die-hard tampon lover, try the Keeper as an alternative. A small rubber cup, the Keeper is inserted in the vagina to catch the blood. Although incredibly environmentally friendly, it shouldn't be used by women at risk of cervical cancer or whose overall health is poor.

Take an Epsom salt bath

An Epsom salt bath is an excellent de-stressor. The magnesium in the salts is an essential mineral for minimising menstrual woes – including PMS, cramping, endometriosis, fibroids. It also helps to oxygenate the body and release toxins. Epsom salt baths are particularly beneficial if you're exposed to a lot of electro magnetic radiation (EMR), for example from computers. If you feel the flu or a cold coming on, also take an Epsom salt bath.

Caution: Because there are so many chemicals in our water today, I would not recommend taking extended baths unless you have at the very minimum a chlorine filter on your bath tap.

Taking the Epsom salt bath

It's particularly beneficial to have regular Epsom salt baths, say two or three a week. If you don't usually have baths, you'll need to build up slowly. Start by taking a bath for five minutes, then ten minutes and so on. Then when you can comfortably sit in a bath for 20 minutes, start adding the Epsom salts.

1 Heat the bath to approximately 40 degrees Celsius. This is a comfortable heat, but enough to cause you to sweat a little.

2 Add 4 to 6 cups of Epsom salts plus a handful of bicarbonate of soda (the latter is optional).

3 Immerse yourself in the tub for at least 20 minutes.

4 Don't shower afterwards.

5 Lie down on your bed or the floor.

6 Cover yourself with towels to maintain your body heat.

7 Lie still for 10 minutes. You will feel a pulsation at the base of your spine which will gradually subside. This is the cerebral spinal fluid being pumped to your brain.

8 Enjoy your new sense of relaxation and vitality!

Take a natural light bath

For a healthy hormonal system, we need natural light in the day and dark at night. Wearing sunglasses also restricts light reception, depleting the eye of vitamin A. To maintain overall wellbeing you need a "natural light bath" every day. We need vitamin D from sunlight for calcium absorption. Calcium is an essential mineral for many body functions. PMS sufferers have been found to be calcium deficient and breast cancer has a strong association with low levels of vitamin D and lack of sunlight (Enig & Fallon, 2001). Calcium also aids peristalsis, eases constipation and, along with magnesium, can minimise menstrual pain.

As a minimum, expose bare arms, neck and face ideally for 30 minutes, between 7.30 to 8.00 am in the southern hemisphere, or between 8.00 am and 8.00 pm during daylight hours in the northern hemisphere. If you can't get a full half hour, at least ten minutes will be beneficial. If it's too cold outside, expose your face only but double the time. Make sure to get extra sunlight on your days off if you work inside. However, avoid prolonged exposure to the sun at midday. Also make sure you're eating a mineral rich diet (see food section) so that you have some calcium in your body to metabolise!

Use castor oil and linseed packs

Recommended for period pain, endometriosis, fibroids, cysts, irregular periods or no period at all, and also constipation, castor oil and linseed packs are also beneficial for the nervous system and the immune system.

Caution: I recommend you **don't** use the packs while you're menstruating, particularly if you bleed heavily.

Making your castor oil pack

You will need:

¼ to ½ cup of castor oil – preferably cold pressed and pesticide free

A piece of cotton or wool flannelette, folded into four thicknesses and large enough to cover your abdomen

A bath towel to lie on

An extra towel, folded, to cover the castor oil pack

Hot water bottle or heating pad

Castor oil pack holder (see Resources)

1. Soak the cotton or flannelette with castor oil. The initial soaking will use up to ½ cup of oil, later soakings will use less as the cloth becomes saturated with the oil. Eventually you can either wash the cloth or throw it away.
2. Place the soaked pad over your abdomen.
3. Put the hot water bottle, or heating pad, in the holder.
4. Place the holder on top of the pad.
5. Strap the holder and pad around your body to hold everything in place.
6. Cover the pack with a folded towel to keep in the heat.
7. Lie still for 30 to 45 minutes – enjoy, bliss out, dream into the experience or, if you are like me, fall in and out of sleep!
8. When you've finished with the pack, store it in the refrigerator.

The packs do take commitment. Start gradually – once a week for about 20 minutes, until you're familiar with its effect on you. Build up to three days in a row and then have a day off. If you're unable to do three days in a row, aim for three times a week. Keep this up for at least three or four months then taper off to once a week. Listen to what your body is telling you and adjust use accordingly.

Making your linseed pack

A little less messy, and cheaper, than castor oil packs, linseed packs don't take long to do.

You will need:

Approximately 1/3 cup organic linseed

Warm filtered or bottled water

A piece of cotton material to cover your abdomen

A bath towel to lie on

1 Grind the linseed using a mortar and pestle. It's important to grind the seeds by hand as some of the healing and nutrient power is lost through electrical grinding.

2 Add enough warm purified water to make a paste.

3 Lying down on the towel, spread the paste over your abdomen.

4 Cover your abdomen with the piece of cotton.

5 Lie still for 15 minutes.

Start gradually – once a week for about 15 minutes, until you are familiar with its effect on you. Build up to three days in a row and then have a day off. If you're unable to do three days in a row, aim for three times a week. Keep this up for at least three or four months then taper off to once a week. Listen to what your body is telling you and adjust use accordingly.

Take care of your breasts

Poorly fitting bras are bad for breast health and may contribute to breast sensitivity. Bras artificially restrict the lymphatic system making it difficult to flush out accumulated wastes from the body. This allows toxins to gather in the breast tissue which forms a breeding ground for a number of health problems including breast cancer (McTaggart, 1996).

Avoid underwiring especially if you work with computers – the metal may act as antennae, focusing electromagnetic radiation around the breast.

A Sydney-based company, Full Bloom, has produced the Bodywise bra. Made without underwires, hooks and eyes or heavy elastic, they accommodate the normal cyclical changes in a woman's breast.

Learn the Deer Exercise

A Taoist exercise that is beneficial for healing menstrual problems, the Deer Exercise builds energy; balances the endocrine system; reduces, and in some cases eliminates period pain; smoothes out the emotional bumpiness of the premenstruum; reduces blood flow; and strengthens the pelvic floor. Additional benefits include increased awareness of your body and even greater intimacy with yourself.

The exercise takes only 7 to 10 minutes a day and involves a gentle massaging of the breasts in a circular motion for a specific number of times. This is followed by a meditation to reabsorb the energy that has been generated into the body and balance the endocrine system. Success builds with regularity of practice.

Lisa Bodley's book *Recreating Menstruation* (see book list for details) has a comprehensive and straightforward description of the Deer Exercise. You can easily learn to do the exercise from her book.

Practise the Buteyko technique

Like good food, correct breathing is essential for all body functions, and improved overall wellbeing will ease menstrual problems. In particular it can balance blood sugar levels, ease depression and menstrual pain and may also help with infertility.

The Buteyko technique is a breathing practice initially used to manage asthma. However, it's an exercise everyone can benefit from, especially anyone who has sinus problems or a tendency to breathe through the mouth.

This is not a technique you can teach yourself from a book – it must be learnt from a trained Buteyko practitioner. Once learnt you have it for a life. I practise the exercise daily to maintain my overall wellbeing and find it especially beneficial.

7 Checklist for Sufferers

Pre Menstrual Syndrome (PMS)

- Be Prepared! *Always* know where you are in the cycle so that you're aware when you're moving into "that time of the month".
- Keep your schedule as light as possible in this phase.
- Plan for some personal space where you don't have to take care of anyone else.
- Do something indulgent, different from usual.
- Eat magnificently – regular meals full of fresh vegetables, fruit and protein (see food section).
- Avoid all soft drinks, refined carbohydrates and other junk food, and all foods with synthetic additives and preservatives.
- Carry wholesome snacks with you for the premenstrual blood sugar swings.
- Bathe in natural light between 7.30 and 8.00 in the morning (for the southern hemisphere) and between 8.00 a.m. and 8.00 p.m. in daylight (for the northern hemisphere).
- Combined with a healthy diet, try a high quality acidophilus supplement and/or digestive enzymes to improve bloating and other digestive complaints.
- See a natural health practitioner to improve digestive function and check for candida.
- To minimise premenstrual headaches, don't skip any meals, avoid alcohol and getting dehydrated.
- Only drink purified or bottled water from glass or clear plastic.
- Slow down – try being less "out there" and become more internal and reflective.
- Use that premenstrual "criticising" energy to clean up things in your life that aren't working for you. See it also as a time for self examination, a "calling to account" moment.

- Crankiness could be a sign you simply need more personal space, or that it's time you spoke out on some things.
- Use that premenstrual vulnerability for some tender, down time.
- If you become vague and forgetful, slow down, let yourself be dreamy. Take more short breaks throughout the day.
- Give Superwoman a day off. Ask for more help!
- Sleep in late, take afternoon naps, go to bed early. Fit in some extra dreaming time if you want to.
- Become interested in your dreams, particularly in the premenstruum as they can sometimes become more powerful and even visionary at this time.
- Notice how your extra sensitivity allows you to be more psychic or intuitive.
- If you work with computers or in an office environment with a lot of electrical equipment, use ionisers (see environment section).
- Avoid excessive use of mobile phones at ***all*** times. I recommend avoiding them altogether, especially during the premenstrual phase.
- Avoid wearing perfumes or strong smelling deodorants/antiperspirants (see environment section).
- Exercise, exercise, exercise! Think of it as an all-month activity. You may find just as you come close to bleeding you might feel less inclined to do it. This is OK, especially if you're exercising regularly.
- Practise the Deer Exercise, fabulous for easing the premenstrual moodiness.
- Take regular Epsom salt baths.
- To ease breast sensitivity, wear healthy bras, or none at all. Also reduce or stop coffee consumption, avoid all deep-fried foods.
- Seek out an understanding counsellor or psychotherapist, particularly if you experience intense depression, feel suicidal or have violent outbursts of rage.

Period Pain

- Clean up your diet – especially eat more fresh vegies and fruit.
- Avoid deep-fried foods and rich fatty foods, particularly just before and during bleeding.
- Try small, easily digestible meals when you're bleeding such as hearty soups with lots of vegetables, a little seaweed, some beans, fish or organic chook.
- Avoid tampons. Consider cloth pads instead.
- Don't use an IUD – if you already have one, consider having it removed.
- Learn about natural fertility management and/or use condoms or a diaphragm for contraception.
- Exercise regularly throughout the month, but ease up when bleeding.
- Do yoga regularly, particularly those poses that strengthen the uterus/ pelvic region – over time your pain will ease.
- Discover shiatsu massage. You can learn movements and massage "points" that will ease pain.
- Get a chiropractor or osteopath to check your body structure.
- Take regular Epsom salt baths.
- Use linseed or castor oil packs throughout the cycle but avoid castor oil packs when bleeding.
- Avoid wheat and unfermented soy products, especially if you have a tendency to constipation. Also eat plenty of mineral rich fresh vegies, seaweed, seeds such as linseed and fruit (especially apricots, figs and prunes).
- Practise the Deer Exercise every day for at least two months.
- Work towards being able to do without drugs – keep them for emergencies. When you take drugs you lose touch with your body and may do inappropriate things, e.g. pushing yourself, eating non-supportive foods.
- If you have to take painkillers, still move gently and kindly with yourself. Just do the best you can.
- Try to arrange your life around the pain so that you can have space when it comes to either rest or do some gentle movement.

- If you have a partner or friend ask them to massage you where you sense you'd like it.
- Using the voice (for example shouting, singing, chanting) can help to ease pain.
- Experiment! Explore the pain. Listen to it. Learn about its characteristics. You may get clues as to what's happening.

Endometriosis

- Follow the strategies in the previous section on "Period Pain".
- Build your immune system. Endometriosis is linked to damage from chemicals and drugs, including fertility drugs, to the immune system.
- The healthy dietary recommendations are a critical foundation for turning endometriosis around.
- Follow the environmental recommendations as closely as possible.
- Nourish yourself at all levels. Take lots of rest, especially at menstruation.
- Find a health practitioner versed in nutritional and natural therapies to help you strengthen and detoxify your body, for example, naturopathy and Traditional Chinese Medicine.
- Remember it's OK to take small steps. Keep going steadily, adding new health strategies as you can manage and afford them. Soon you'll notice wellbeing spreading through you like a delicious atmosphere.

Fibroids and Cysts

- Follow the dietary recommendation closely. Avoiding dairy products, for at least three months has proved successful in some cases.
- Try a fairly vigorous exercise programme.
- Follow the environmental recommendations as closely as possible.
- Use linseed or castor oil packs at least three times a week on the abdomen and maintain a programme for at least three months.
- Consider regular clay packs on the abdomen. Clay is famous for its healing properties and in particular its ability to draw toxins from the body.
- Take regular Epsom salt baths.

- If you're close to the end of your menstruating years, remember that fibroids naturally decrease with menopause.
- Practise the Deer Exercise regularly.
- Watch for stress – de-stress your life.
- Try naturopathy and Traditional Chinese Medicine.

Heavy Bleeding

- Top of the list is clean up your diet. Especially avoid all junk foods, synthetic colourings and additives.
- Follow the environmental recommendations closely.
- Avoid tampons – consider using cloth pads. Some women have commented that their bleeding has decreased just with the use of the cloth pads.
- Practise the Deer Exercise regularly.
- Make sure you're well rested.
- Give yourself two to three cycles for benefits of the above to kick in.
- Seek professional help if none of these practices make a difference.

Lack of a Period

- If you haven't had a period for a few months, seek professional guidance.
- Because this can sometimes occur from stress and eating disorders, get support for these issues.
- Follow the food guidelines carefully and include organic dairy products.
- Be kind to yourself! Try some soothing massage.
- Try castor oil or linseed packs.
- Hot baths (fling in some Epson salts for good measure) sometimes help to bring on a period that is a little late.
- Practise the Deer Exercise.

Finding Meaning

Depth of meaning comes from your capacity to "feel into" an experience rather than just intellectualising about it. This will develop with time. Here are some useful questions and suggestions to get you going. Write freely in response to them.

- What would I love to do premenstrually and at menstruation if I didn't have to worry about others?
- What am I confronted with premenstrually? What is upsetting?
- What am I confronted with as I bleed/am in pain?
- If my endometriosis/fibroid/cyst had a voice, what would it say to me?
- What do I need emotionally?
- Am I honouring my creative voice? If not, what would I need to do to honour my creativity?
- How easy am I with my body?
- If I had the courage to speak my truth, what would I like to say? This might be to your partner, friends, or at work. Or it might be something more public about what's happening in your community or the world. If you don't feel ready to speak out, write down your feelings, or role play them.

Try drawing, using clay, or making music to represent your symptoms. Take some quiet space and time to tune into your experience of your symptoms and then pick up the medium you choose to work with. Let the internal experiences flow without censoring them. Remember, this is not about creating a work of art!

It's sometimes useful to share observations with others. In speaking about your ideas you may find they become clearer.

Delicious Healing Recipes

Homemade remedies using everyday food items are a wonderful non-toxic and inexpensive way to support overall wellbeing and ease menstrual problems. Make them a part of your daily routine.

Nettle Brew

Surprisingly tasty, this mineral rich drink is a great tonic.

Benefits

- *excellent for strengthening kidneys and adrenals*
- *pick-me-up if you're fatigued*
- *stabilises blood sugar levels*
- *promotes healthy bones*
- *helps ease cramping and profuse menstrual flow.*

The American herbalist and author Susan Weed speaks of nettle as a wonderful ally for women. She claims that two cups of nettle infusion daily will nourish and stabilise energy in the reproductive/hormonal systems, build nutrient rich blood and expand the cells' capacity to metabolise nutrients (Weed, 1989).

You will need:

A couple of handfuls of dried organic, or fresh, nettle

1 litre of boiling filtered water

Place the nettle into a lidded container. Add the boiling water and allow to steep for four hours. Drink the brew over one or two days and refrigerate unused portion. Nettle brew is a delicious drunk hot or cold – but don't drink it ice cold. If you don't have time to brew the nettle, make it the same way as you would a herb tea – just steep the leaves in boiling water for a few minutes.

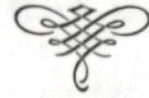

Ginger Tea

Benefits

- *aids digestion*
- *eases menstrual cramping and nausea*
- *helpful if your periods have stopped temporarily*
- *pick-me-up during the premenstrual tired phase.*

You will need:

A small quantity of fresh ginger

Enough filtered or bottled water for one cup of tea

Finely grate the ginger (about a teaspoon). Add hot water and allow to steep for a few minutes. Alternatively cut some slices of ginger and simmer covered for 5 minutes.

Miso Soup (for one)

Miso soup, like the ubiquitous chicken soup, is a panacea for all ills! Miso can be added to any soup or stew as seasoning, or you can try the following simple recipe. Include plenty of seaweed and you have an even more nourishing brew.

Benefits

- *strengthening and alkalising properties*
- *helps the body resist disease*
- *full of lactobacillus (the same as in yogurt) to aid digestion and assimilation of vitamins and minerals (as long as you don't boil it)*
- *promotes long life and good health*
- *treats and prevents radiation sickness*
- *neutralises some of the effects of smoking and air pollution.*

You will need:

A handful of vegetables, e.g. daikon (a long white radish), Chinese greens, pumpkin, carrots, green beans

1 inch strip of kombu, wakame or Tasmanian float leaf seaweed

Miso (brown rice miso or barley miso are good ones for soup)

A grating of ginger and/or shallots to garnish

One bowl of filtered or bottled water

Wash the seaweed and chop the vegies. Place the vegetables and seaweed in a pot with enough water for one bowl of soup. Bring to boil and simmer covered until the vegetables are just cooked. Remove the seaweed and cut it into thin strips. Return the strips to the pot. Put approximately half to three quarters of a teaspoon of miso into the bowl – experiment with the amount until you find the flavour you like. Add grated ginger and/or chopped shallots with a little of the hot liquid to form a paste. Then add the rest of the soup.

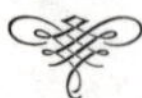

Miso in a hurry

Miso soup is a great way to start the day, especially in the premenstruum. If you're in a hurry, simply boil water and add to the miso for a miso drink. You can enhance this by adding a little grated ginger/chopped shallots/ nori seaweed/crushed garlic. Delicious!

Caution: *If you suffer from candida albicans (yeast overgrowth) and similar fungal infections, use miso sparingly. Like other fermented foods, miso absorbs toxins from plastic containers, so store it in a glass, enamel or wood container (Pitchford, 1993).*

Soup stock

Yet another mineral brew – especially for those of you who are having trouble getting excited about seaweeds and enjoy eating a little meat and fish.

Make stock from the bones of meat or fish by covering the bones with water, bringing to the boil and then simmering on a low heat for approximately 20 minutes. Towards the end of simmering time add a teaspoon of cider vinegar. The acidity of the vinegar will draw the minerals from the bones.

Lemon Water

Lemon water is one of those all-purpose remedies, which everyone can enjoy – always keep some prepared.

Benefits

- *supports the liver*
- *aids digestion.*

You will need:

One organic lemon

Two cups of filtered or bottled water

Roughly chop the lemon and place in a lidded glass container, such as a glass jar (the container ***must*** *be glass). Add two cups of filtered or bottled water and allow to stand for two hours in the refrigerator before drinking.*

Drink approximately a third of a cup after each meal and enjoy it at other times of the day too – especially if you're on a detoxification program. Drink a glass when you get up and your liver will be singing for the rest of the day! Also drink if you've been in polluted environments or feel a flu or cold coming on.

Rejuvelac

Rejuvelac is a fermented drink made from wheat sprouts. You can drink it straight or use it to make seed and nut cheeses and other ferments.

Benefits

- *cleans the system*
- *improves the condition of the intestinal flora*
- *aids digestion and assimilation of vitamins and mineral.*

You will need:

One cup of wheat grains

Nine cups of bottled or filtered water

First soaking: to one cup of wheat grains add three cups of bottled or filtered water and allow to stand for 48 hours (in hot weather this time can be reduced to 36 hours). Pour off the liquid.

Second, third and fourth soaking: use the same wheat grains. Add two cups of bottled or filtered water and soak for 24 hours. Pour off liquid after each soaking.

Rejuvelac should taste quite sweet, not sour. If it tastes unpleasant it's probably over-fermented.

One cup of wheat grains will yield approximately 9 cups of rejuvelac. Refrigerate rejuvelac that you don't use immediately. It will keep in the refrigerator for up to five days. After soakings you can eat the wheat grains, put them into bread or sow them to grow wheat grass.

Source: Kenton, S. and L. (1984) *Raw Energy*, London: Vermilion.

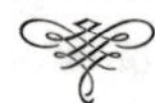

Finding Extra Help

Therapies and health organisations

Australia

To find a qualified practitioner in your area, contact:

Association of Remedial Masseurs, 1/20 Blaxland Road, Ryde, NSW 2112; Ph: (02) 9807 4769

Australian Acupuncture Association, PO Box 5142, West End, Qld 4101; Ph: (07) 3846 5866

Association of Massage Therapists (NSW) PO Box 1248, Bondi Junction NSW 1355; Ph: (02) 9300 9405

Australian Association of Reflexology, 2 Stewart St, Matraville, NSW 2036; Ph: (02) 9311 2322

Australian Hypnotherapists Association, FREECALL 1800 067 557

Australian Institute of Homoeopathy, 29 Bertram St, Chatswood, NSW 2067; Ph: (02) 9415 3928

Australian Natural Therapists Association, PO Box A964, Sydney, NSW 2000; Ph: (02) 9283 2234; country and interstate 1800 817 577

Australian Music Therapy Association, PO Box 79, Turramurra, NSW, 2074; Ph: (02) 9449 5279; Email: information@austmta.org.au

Australian Osteopathic Association, PO Box 6999, Turramurra, NSW 2074; Ph: (02) 9449 4799

Australian Society of Clinical Hypnotherapists, 30 Denistone Rd, Eastwood, NSW 2122; Ph: (02) 9874 2776

Australasian Society of Oral Medicine and Toxicology (ASOMAT), PO Box A860, Sydney South, NSW 2000; Ph: (02) 9867 1111, Fax: (02) 9283 2230 (for safe removal of dental amalgam)

Australian Traditional Medicine Society, PO Box 1027, Meadowbank, NSW 2114; Ph: (02) 9809 6800

Buteyko Institute www.bibh.org. Australian contacts: Roger Price at www.buteykoabc.com or Ph: 1800 777 798; Freida Belakhova

Ph: (02) 9553 7118.

Chiropractors Association of Australia, FREECALL 1800 803 665.

O'Keefe Health and Education Group Pty Ltd (Clinical Hypnotherapy/counselling-practitioners/training), 27 Meymott St, Randwick, NSW 2031. Ph: (02) 9326 6603 or 0403 398 808. Fax: (02) 9399 6587, Email: info@tracieokeefe.com, Website: www.tracieokeefe.com

Psychotherapy and Counselling Federation of Australia (PACFA), PO Box 481, Carlton South, Victoria 3053; Ph: (03) 9639 8330, Fax: (03) 9639 8340, Email: PACFA@bigpond.com, Website: www.pacfa.org.au

Shiatsu Therapy Association of Australia, 332 Carlisle St, Balaclava, Vic 3183; Ph: (03) 9530 0067; PO Box 47, Waverley, NSW 2024; Ph: (02) 9314 5248

New Zealand

Association of NZ Ortho-Bionomists Inc. PO Box 31-060, Milford, Auckland.

New Zealand Association of Therapeutic Massage Practitioners. PO Box 375, Hamilton. Email: nzatmp@ihug.co.nz

New Zealand Charter of Health Practitioners Inc. PO Box 36588, Northcote, Auckland. Phone: 094436255. Umbrella organisation for all natural therapies.

New Zealand Register of Acupuncturists Inc. PO Box 9950, Wellington. Phone: 0800228786. Email: nzra@acupuncture.org.nz

South Pacific Association of Natural Therapists. 28 Willow Avenue, Birkenhead, Auckland. Ph/fax: (09) 4809089.

United Kingdom

British Association of Counsellors, 1 Regent Place, Rugby, Warwickshire CV21 2PJ

Ph: 01788578328, email: bac@bac.co.uk, website: www.counselling.co.uk

British Chiropractic Association, Blagrave House, 17 Blagrave St, Reading RG1 IQB, Ph: 01189505950. www.chiropractic-uk.co.uk

General Council of Naturopathy, Goswell House, 2 Goswell Rd, Somerset BA16 OJG, Ph: 01458 840072. www.naturopathy.org.uk

General Council of Osteopathy, Osteopathy House, 176 Tower Bridge Rd, London SE1 3OU, Ph: 0207 357 6655

Society of Homoeopaths, 4a Artizan Rd, Northampton NN1 4HN, Ph: 01604621400. www.homeopathy-soh.org

USA

The American Association of Naturopathic Physicians, PO Box 20386, Seattle, WA 98112. Ph: (206) 298-0125

The American Holistic Medical Association, 6728 Old McLean Village, Dr McLean, VA 22101. Ph: (703) 556-9245

Women's business

Alexandra Pope
PO Box 1018,
Bondi Junction, NSW 1355.
Ph/fax: (02) 9310 0591
email: aepope@ozemail.com.au

I offer counselling and psychotherapy for individuals and couples, as well as workshops and one-on-one sessions on menstrual health and menopause. Phone consultations are also available.

Amrita Hobbs
PO Box 337
Kyogle NSW 2474
Ph: 0419 336 291
email: amritahobbs@bigpond.com
www.skyfamily.com/rediscovering-rites

Amrita runs workshops in Australia and overseas to support girls and women through key life passages. Current programs include: Girls Growing Up (mother and daughter, and father and daughter programs); Rites of Passage (for teenagers); Reclaiming First Rites (for women); and Wise Woman healing, a certificated training program.

Felicity Oswell
PO Box 206
Manly, NSW, 1655
Australia
Ph: (02) 9983 9440
email: felwm@ihug.com.au

Felicity, creator of the Wombmoon Calendar, regularly runs Mandala Moon workshops in Australia and Japan using art and dance. She also leads and teaches the Mandala Dance of the 21 Taras and develops Wisdom Moon programs for women focusing on cyclic and menstrual awareness.

Jane Bennett
PO Box 786
Castlemaine, Vic 3450
Australia
Ph: (03) 5472 4922

Jane runs A Blessing Not a Curse workshops for mothers of daughters from 8 to 12 years old to prepare them for menarche.

Katherine Cunningham
Ph: 02 5155 4311
email: living_gently@hotmail.com

Katherine runs menstrual workshops for girls and women on accessing menstrual power through ritual and daily practical tools.

Dr Karin Cutter, PhD
PO Box 5355
Port Macquarie NSW 2444
Ph: 02 6583 2961

Karin is a biochemist, naturopath, homoeopath, herbalist and nutritionist. She provides consultation by telephone and letter if you do not live in the area and are unable to see her in person.

Natural Fertility Management
The Jocelyn Centre
1/46 Grosvenor Centre
Woollahra
NSW 2025
Ph: (02) 9369 2047, Fax: (02) 9369 5179
website: www.fertility.com.au
National Coordinator: Jane Bennett

This centre offers private consultations and a correspondence service for contraception, conscious conception and overcoming fertility problems. They also provide a range of medical and holistic therapies for reproductive and general health issues.

The International College of Spiritual Midwifery
The Balcony Room, Level 1, 210 Lonsdale St,
Melbourne, Vic 3000.
Ph/fax: (03) 9654 3737

Offer a range of seminars, workshops, and individual sessions on ancient women's knowledge in a modern context: fertility, conscious conception, childbirth preparation, spiritual midwifery, healing, women's mysteries retreats, adolescent programs and much more.

Wise Woman Business Pty Ltd
Kerry Hampton
Fertility Awareness and Menstrual Cycle Education

Kerry offers individual or couple tuition, women only groups, distance education, and mother and daughter evenings.
PO Box 250 Canterbury Vic 3126; ph/fax: (03) 9830 5280

Women's Wilderness Quests
Maggie Mackenzie,
PO Box 42, Clovelly West, NSW 2031
(02) 9664 1968

Maggie, a psychotherapist, holds vision quests in pristine wilderness, including a three day solo, with full support and community. Quests offer a deeper connection with nature, self and life direction. They are also used to mark life's transitions.

New Zealand

Luna Collective for Women's Wellness
PO Box 836
Nelson
Ph/fax: (03) 5458505
Email: lunacollective@ts.co.nz
Website: www.luna.tasman.net

This collective is non-profit and promotes women's health, in particular menstrual health. It produces information sheets and has menstruation and fertility resources.

Natural Fertility Management
Jo Barnet
220c Kilmore St, Christchurch.
Ph: (03) 365 1906.
Email: herbald@xtra.co.nz

The Health Alternatives for Women (THAW)
PO Box 884
Christchurch
Phone: (03) 796970 Fax: (03) 663470 Email: thaw@ch.planet.gen.nz

A health information and resource centre offering a variety of health services.

United Kingdom

Cabby Laffy
Ph: 020 7482 6371
email: cabbylaffy@yahoo.co.uk

Cabby offers one-on-one and couple counselling sessions as well as group sessions and workshops on fertility and/or sexuality, providing practical and emotional support.

Natural Fertility Management
Carla Halford
1 Grove Cottage
Longnor, Shropshire, SY57PS
Ph/fax: 017 43718 951.
Email: carla@zesty.com

Women and Health
4 Carol St,
Camden Town, London NW1.
Ph: 020 7482 2786
Resources and women's centre offering low cost complementary therapies.

USA

Ash Tree Publishing and the Wise Woman Centre
Susun Weed
PO Box 64 Woodstock
NY 12498.
Phone: (914) 246-8081

This centre provides classes, books, phone consultations.

Dr Christiane Northrup
PO Box 199
Yarmouth, Maine 04096
USA
(800) 804 0935
website: www.DrNorthrup.com

Medical practitioner and well known author, Dr Northrup also produces a newsletter, information tapes and women's health videos.

Menstrual Health Foundation
Tamara Slayton
708 Gravenstein Hwy North PMB #181
Sebastopol, California 95472
Ph: 707 522 8662, Fax: 707 823 2137
www.cyclesinc.org
www.e-irmc.org

Tamara offers educational programs on coming of age, menstruation and fertility cycles, menopause, teacher training, curriculum development and program design.

Mysteries of Life
Judith Barr
PO Box 218, North Salem, New York, 10560.
Ph/fax: 914-669-5822.
Email: judbarr@judithbarr.com
Website: www.judithbarr.com

Judith works with individuals and groups worldwide. She teaches on the feminine and women's mysteries, including workshops on menstruation, menopause and sexuality.

Natural Fertility Management
National coordinator (USA): Joyce Stahmann
Email: stahmann@yahoo.com
Website: www.herbalwellness.net

Orthobionomy
Zoee Crowley
1023 Makamua Street
Wailuku, Hawaii, 96793
Ph/fax: 8082429168
Email: zoee@maui.net
Website: www.maui.net/-zoee

Zoee is an orthobionomy practitioner who also trains orthobionomists worldwide.

Australia

The Original Moonphase Period Piece (cloth pads)
PO Box 1018, Bondi Junction, NSW 1355; ph/fax: (02) 9310 0591
email: aepope@ozemail.com.au

Rad Pads (cloth pads)
PO Box 786, Castlemaine Vic. 3450. Ph: (03) 5472 4922, Fax: (03) 5470 5766
email: enquiries@fertility.com.au

Wise Woman Cloths (organic cloth pads)
PO Box 250, Canterbury, Vic 3126; ph/fax: (03) 9830 5280

Wemoon (cloth pads)
PO Box 249 Byron Bay, NSW 2481; ph: (02) 6684 6300

The Keeper
PO Box 610, Harbord, NSW 2096
email: keepercup@hotmail.com
www.morning.com.au/go/keeper

Sea sponges are available from selected health food stores and pharmacies.

Organic tampons are available in many health food stores.

New Zealand

Moontime Aotearoa
email: lunacollective@ts.co.nz
Website: www.luna.tasman.net

Also available in most health food shops around New Zealand.

The Keeper
PO Box 47820
Ponsonby
Auckland

Sea Sponges
Maree Hassick
Waiora Mara
Pokororo, RD 1
Motueka
Phone: 03 5268829

United Kingdom

Ecofemme UK
Dominique Pahud
17 Talbot Road
Knowle, Bristol, BS42NE
Phone: 0117 904 9726

Feminine Alternatives
18 Tor View Avenue, Glastonbury, Somerset
BA6 8AF.
Ph: 01458 834787
Menstrual pads, sponges, fertility information.

USA

Cascade Healthcare Products, Inc.
Moonflower Natural Products Catalogue (cloth pads)
141 Commercial St. NE, Salem, OR 97301.
Ph: (503) 371-445; Fax: (503) 371-5395, orders 1 800-443-9942.
www.1CASCADE.com.

Gladrags
PO Box 12648, Portland, OR 97212
Ph: (503) 282-0436, 1-800-799-GLAD
email: b@gladrags.com

Menstrual Health Foundation (cloth pads)
708 Gravenstein Hwy North PMB #181
Sebastopol, California 95472
Ph: 707 522 8662, Fax: 707 823 2137
www.cyclesinc.org
www.e-irmc.org

Japan

Cloth pads

Nawa Prasad, 3-15-3, Nishi Ogi Minami, Suginami-Ku, Tokyo 167 - 0053
Ph: (03) 3332 1187, Fax: (03) 3331 3067
Also contact point for women's workshops run by Felicity Oswell (see under Women's business)

Nanohana, 22-75 Sekitacho, Tanaka, Sakyo - Ku, Kyoto City 606 - 8203
Ph: (075) 711 8264, Fax: (075) 711 5584

Ways Ltd, 57-B1F-A Sanjou Takakura Higashi Iru, Nakagyouku, Kyoto
604-8111. Ph: (075) 417-3546, Fax: (075) 417-3545
Website: www.ways.co.jp

Healing products

Australia

Full Bloom Pty Ltd
PO Box 393, Paddington, NSW 2021.
Ph: (02) 9361 6052, 1800 068 870. Email: bodywise@fullbloom.com.au
Website: www.fullbloom.com.au
Comfortable and attractive bras and underwear for women of all shapes and sizes including pregnant women and nursing mothers. Also leopard skin undies with red gusset to wear at menstruation!

Aironic Pty Ltd
PO Box 216
Lane Cove NSW 2066.
Ph: (02) 9439 7599
Ionisers for home and car (worth getting especially if your health is poor and/or you do a lot of driving).

Pesticide-free castor oil and pack holder
You may find these at selected health practitioners or you can import your own from The Heritage Store, USA (see below).

USA

Avena Botanicals
219 Mill St
Rockport, Maine 04856.
Ph: (207) 594-0694

Women owned and run, this organisation provides organic herbs and products, classes and cloth pads.

Cascade Healthcare Products, Inc.
Moonflower Natural Products Catalogue (herbs and products for babies and women) and the Birth and Life Bookstore Catalogue
141 Commercial St. NE, Salem, OR 97301.
Ph: (503) 371-445, Fax: (503) 371-5395, orders 1 800-443-9942.
www.1CASCADE.com

Mountain Rose Herbs
20818 High St
North San Juan, CA 95960.
Ph: 800-879-3337.
Website: www.botanical.com/mtrose
This company will ship internationally.

The Heritage Store
Dept C,
PO Box 444
Virginia Beach, VA 23458-0444, USA.
Ph: 757 428 4941, Fax: 757 428 3632.
Email: heritage@caycecures.com
Supply pesticide-free castor oil and pack holder.

Support groups and organisations

Australia

DES (diethylstilboestrol) support – PO Box 282, Camberwell, Vic 3124, Phone: 03 9870 0536 and 14 Edmundson Close, Thornleigh, NSW 2120, Phone: 02 9875 4820

Endometriosis Complementary Therapies Support Group, Lorraine Henderson, Ph: 0418 177 951

Endometriosis Support Group, Royal Hospital for Women, Barker St, Randwick, NSW 2031 Ph: 9382 6700

Endometriosis Association NSW, Hemsley House, 20 Roslyn St, Potts Point, NSW 2011; Ph: (02) 9356 0450, Fax: (02) 9357 2334

Endometriosis Association VIC, 37 Andrew Cres, South Croydon, Vic 3136

Endometriosis Support Group QLD, Penny Fenton, Ph: (07) 5502 0166 (W) 0402 020061 (mobile)

Women's Community Health Centres – check telephone directory or state government health department for a centre in you area

Women's Health Victoria (03) 9662 3755. Health Information Line: (03) 9662 3742. Email: whv@whv.org.au. Website: www.whv.org.au

New Zealand

DES (diethylstilboestrol) support. Prof. Charlotte Paul, Preventative and Social Medicine, Otago Medical School, Box 913, Dunedin.

New Zealand Endometriosis Foundation. PO Box 1683, Palmerston North, Ph/fax 06 3592613. Email: nzendo@xtra.co.nz Website: www.nzendo.co.nz

United Kingdom

DES (diethylstilboestrol) support – c/- NWCI, 16-20 South Cumberland St, Dublin 2.
DES (diethylstilboestrol) support – c/- Women's Health (see below).
Endometriosis Society Helpline, 02072222776
National Association for Premenstrual Syndrome
7 Swift's Ct, High St, Seal, Kent TN15 OEG.
PO Box 72, Sevenoaks, Kent TN13 1XQ
Ph/fax: 01732760011. Helpline: 01732760012
Email: naps@charity.vfree.com. Website: www.pms.org.uk

The Menopause Helpline Ltd
228 Muswell Hill Broadway, London N10 3SH.
Ph: 0181 4445202, Fax: 0181 444 6442
Offers support for women suffering from side effects of HRT and the Pill.

Women's Health
52 Featherstone St,
London EC1Y 8RT.
Ph: 020 7251 6580
www.womenshealthlondon.org.uk
A resource, information and support centre.

United States

DES (diethylstilboestrol) support – US National Office, 610 -16th St #301, Oakland, CA 94612 Ph: 1-800-DES-9288 or (510) 465 4011. Fax: (510) 465 4815. Email: desact@well.sf.ca.us

Canada

DES (diethylstilboestrol) support – National Office, 5890 Monkland, Suite 203, Montreal, Quebec H4A 1G2

Websites

www.laraowen.com

www.menstruation.com.au

www.endometriosisassn.org

Environmentally friendly organisations

Australia

Chemfree Cleaning
C/- Cleanhouse Effect
445 King Street, Newtown, NSW
Mobile: 0403 179819

Cleanhouse Effect shops (Planet Ark)
445 King St, Newtown, NSW
37 Cantonment Street, Fremantle, WA

Enviro-Tru
14 Mort Street, Katoomba NSW
Phone: 02 47825375, Email: azura@pnc.com.au
Offers mail order service for environmentally friendly cleaning products.

Systems Pest Management
1/27a Oxford St, Epping, NSW
Ph: (02) 9865 3153.
This company provides alternative pest extermination and has strict standards. If you don't live in their area, speak to them for guidance or check the internet, your local environment centre or health food shop.

Total Environment Centre
Level 2, 362 Kent St
Sydney NSW 2000
Ph: (02) 9299 5599, Fax: (02) 9299 4411.
Website: www.tec.ncccnsw.org.au

Working Women's Centre
157 Wardell Street, Dulwich Hill, NSW
Phone: 02 95595355

National Occupational Health and Safety Commission
92 Parramatta Rd, Camperdown, NSW
Phone: (02) 9577 9555
Website: www.nohsc.gov.au

United Kingdom

Women's Environmental Network
PO Box 30626,
London E1 1TZ.
Ph: 020 7481 9004. Email: wenuk@gn.apc.org
Website: www.gn.apc.org/wen

Organically grown produce

Australia

Mooneys
PO Box 352
Port Macquarie NSW 2444
Phone: 02 65837883
Fax: 02 65832235

If you have difficulty finding organic food locally, Mooneys deliver biodynamic and organic produce around Australia free with a minimum order.

The National Association for Sustainable Agriculture, Australia (NASAA)
Head Office: PO Box 768
Stirling, SA, 5152
Ph: (08) 370 8455, Fax: (08) 370 8381

This association will help you find a supplier in your area.

Australian Gen-ethics Network
c/o 340 Gore Hill
Fitzroy, Vic 3065
Ph: (03) 9416 2222

Provides information about genetic engineering and genetically modified food.

New Zealand

BIOGRO
PO Box 9693
Marion Square
Wellington
Phone: (04) 8019741
Fax: (04) 8019742
Email: info@bio-gro.co.nz

Fairground Eco Store
PO Box 91718
AMSC
Auckland
Ph/fax: (09) 3768577 or 0800773247

Provides mail order service.

Soil and Health Association
PO Box 36170
Northcote
Auckland
Ph/fax: (09) 4804440
Email: soil@health.pl.net

United Kingdom

The Soil Association
Bristol House
40-46 Victoria Street
Bristol, BS16BY
Ph: 01179290661
Website: www.soilassociation.org.uk
Provides a directory of organic food suppliers in your area.

References

Best S. (2000) 'Microwave Ovens' in *What Doctors Don't Tell You*, Vol 10, No. 12, 2000.

Enig, M. & Fallon, S. 'The Whole Fat, and Nothing But' in *What Doctors Don't Tell You*, Vol 12, No. 1, 2000.

McTaggart, L. (1996) 'Bring Back the Bra Burner' in *What Doctors Don't Tell You*, Vol 7, No. 1, 1996.

Naish, F. and Roberts, J. (1996) *Better Babies: Preconception Care for Prospective Parents,* Sydney: Random House.

Thomas, P. 'Toxic Toiletries' in *What Doctors Don't Tell You*, Vol 10, No. 7, 1999.

Further Reading

More on the amazing world of menstruation

Grahn, J. (1993) *Blood, Bread and Roses: How Menstruation Created the World.* Boston: Beacon Press.

Gray, M. (1994) *Red Mood: Understanding and Using the Gifts of the Menstrual Cycle*. Brisbane: Element Books Ltd.

Owen, L. (1998) *Honouring Menstruation: A Time of Self Renewal.* Freedom: Crossing Press.

Pope, A. (2001) *The Wild Genie: The Healing Power of Menstruation*. Bowral: Sally Milner Publishing.

Shuttle, P. and Redgrove, P. (1989) *The Wise Wound.* London: Paladin.

Shuttle, P., and Redgrove, P. (1995) *Alchemy for Women: Personal Transformation Through Dreams and the Female Cycle.* London: Rider.

Some really healthy books

Ameisen, P. (1997) *Every Breath You Take*, Vic: Cheryl Hingley, 1997.

Angier, N. (1999) *Woman: An Intimate Geography.* London: Virago.

Bays, B. (1999) *The Journey: Extraordinary Guide to Healing Life and Setting Yourself Free*. London: Thorsons.

Bodley, L. (1995) *Recreating Menstruation.* Melbourne: Gnana Foundation (only available from PO Box 246, Yarra Junction, Victoria 3797, Australia. Email: lisa@gnanayoga.com.au)

Epstein, S. and Steinman, D. (1997) *The Breast Cancer Prevention Program.* New York: Macmillan.

Kirner, J. and Rayner, M. (1999) *The Woman's Power Handbook.* Ringwood: Penguin.

Krohn, J., Taylor, Frances A. and Prosser J. (1996) *The Whole Way to Natural Detoxification: The Complete Guide to Clearing Your Body of Toxins.* Point Roberts: Hartley and Marks Publishing Inc.

Lark, S.M. (1984) *PMS: Premenstrual Syndrome Self Help Book.* Berkeley: Celestial Arts.

Leyden-Rubenstein, L.A. (1998) *The Stress Management Handbook: Strategies for Health and Inner Peace.* New Canaan: Keats Publishing Inc.

Naish, F. (1991) *Natural Fertility.* Burra Creek: Sally Milner Publishing.

Naish, F. and Roberts, J. (1996) *The Natural Way to Better Babies: Preconception Health Care for Prospective Parents.* Sydney: Random House.

Northrup, C. (1995) *Women's Bodies, Women's Wisdom.* London: Piatkus.

Pitchford, P. (1993) *Healing with Whole Foods.* Berkeley: North Atlantic Books.

Trickey, R. (1998) *Women, Hormones and The Menstrual Cycle: Herbal and Medical Solutions from Adolescence to Menopause.* St Leonards: Allen & Unwin.

Trickey, R. and Cooke, K. (1998) *Women's Trouble: Natural and Medical Solutions.* St Leonards: Allen & Unwin.

Weed, S (1989) *Healing Wise.* Woodstock: Ash Tree Publishing.

Weed, S. (1992) *Menopausal Years: The Wise Woman Way, Alternative Approaches for Women 30-90.* Woodstock: Ash Tree Publishing.

What Doctors Don't Tell You, Satellite House, 2 Salisbury Rd, London, SW19 4EZ. Email: wddty@zoo.co.uk. Website: www.wddty.co.uk (an informed, useful monthly health publication).

Healthy environments

Baggs, S. and Baggs, J. (1996) *The Healthy House: Creating a Safe, Healthy and Environmentally Friendly Home*, Sydney: HarperCollins Publishers.

Dadd, D.L. (1997) *Home Safe Home: Protecting Yourself and Your Family from Everyday Toxics and Harmful Household Products.* New York: Jeremy P. Tarcher/Putnam.

Both the above books have excellent resource lists.